I0696611

HOW TO MAKE LOVE TO A MAN

Rediscover Sexual Bliss a Close-Up Guide to Safe and Sexy Intimacy, Offering 40 Expert Tips for Healthy and Pleasurable Arousal

Gabrielle Thomas

Copyright © 2023 by Gabrielle Thomas

All rights reserved. No part of this publication may be reproduced, distributed, or transmitted in any form or by any means, including photocopying, recording, or other electronic or mechanical methods, without the prior written permission of the publisher, except in the case of brief quotations embodied in critical reviews and certain other noncommercial uses permitted by copyright law.

Table of contents

Introduction

You may be having sex for the first time or have been having sex for a long time. You might have had a huge number of partners, a few, or perhaps just one. Regardless of your previous sex experiences, knowing how to make love to a man might be the difference between having a mind-blowing romp in the sheets and having vanilla or acceptable sex.

Is it possible to make love and have sex at the same time?
Yes, it most surely is!

This is one way of looking at it. You may have a fancy nine-course meal or simply microwave Macaroni and cheese. They both satisfy your hunger, but a lavish supper with several courses tastes somewhat different, doesn't it?
You can always have sex if all you want is penetration, but making love to a man is about waking all of your senses, delaying satisfaction, appreciating every second

of it, and magnifying and experiencing pleasure to the maximum.

knowing how to make love to a man requires knowing how everyone experiences sexual pleasure differently. One element, however, remains constant: the desire to make your beloved happy.

There are several benefits to learning how to make love to a guy, whether it's your marriage or a one-night fling. It will not only make him incredibly thankful and envious of your sexual skills, but it will also make you enjoy sex a lot more!

The secret to making love passionately

It is true what they say: "The woman only needs to show up and get naked; the guy is under so much pressure." That alone would make any man happy.
But if that's all you do, everything will get stale, much like stale bread after a week. It is despised by everyone.

To keep the fire burning bright, make sure you treat him the same way he treats you. Women are also capable of being powerful and forceful.

It is now OK to have no clue what you are doing or how to continue. Being self-assured is appealing, and chances are he will laugh at your mistakes. You can get over practically everything, so don't be afraid to ruin the mood.

How to make a man cry lustfully while making love to him!

So, how can you have the finest sex you've ever had with your boyfriend while making him weep just thinking about it? Use these tips for the best, most amazing, earth-shattering sex!

CHAPTER 1

1. Talk To Him

The key to being a good lover is effective communication. How would you know what works for your boyfriend if you don't ask him about his wants, desires, and wildest fantasies? Guys are not all alike. Your ex may have loved it when you nibbled his ears, but your present spouse may find it strange, ticklish, or unpleasant.

Remember that discussing sex does not have to be forced or judgmental.

Grab a bottle of wine, sit back, and tell some tales. Alternatively, the next time you're in the bedroom, just ask him, "Do you like it when I do this?" "Should I speed up or slow down?" You'll gain the knowledge you need to better your sex with each other.

2. Avoid being a prude – Everyone despises a prude.

The core of making love is exploring and doing something private with someone personal. It's more than just having sex these days; it's about sharing your feelings with one another and receiving the same degree of communication in return.

Prudence during this time means that you are limited, disconnected, and constricted. This implies that you should endeavor to be open-minded rather than forcing yourself to do something you don't want to do.

3. He's more than his penis.

Men are first and foremost picky about their partner. Everyone is aware of this. They seem to be obsessed with it, regardless of how uninteresting it is. Despite their belief that it is little, it is still their penis.

However, a man is more than his penis. Keep your hats on—it's hard to believe, but there's a man all around that penis. And his balls, to be honest.

Resist the impulse to go straight for his dick, no matter how much he begs you to. The tease is what makes it so entertaining. He'll be harsh when you ultimately move south, so don't go just yet.

4. Sexy zones are also available for men.

All males, like women, have erogenous zones. Examine his body to see what he likes; maybe he likes it when you kiss his fingers, neck, ears, or Adam's apple. Alternatively, if you're feeling very daring, you may try placing your finger in his buttocks or teabagging him! Nothing is sacred after sex, so go ahead and experiment with your love life!

Put on something sensuous, lower the lights, and slowly and softly explore these spots with your hands, lips, and tongue.

5. Retake command

Men are often seen as the dominant gender in sexual encounters. However, it is occasionally necessary to switch things up. So why not be brave and take charge of the situation?

Come upon him, instruct him exactly what to do, throw him against the wall, tie him up, and so on to spice up the bedroom.

Allow your imagination to run wild, and he'll quickly realize what a terrific sex vixen you are.

CHAPTER 2

6. Learn to be submissive when making love to a man.

Allowing your lover to take control and being submissive, on the other hand, may be really appealing. Allow him to hold your hands above your head, help you into different positions, and maybe give you a little paddling now and again.

Encouraging him to take entire control will make him feel powerful and manly, and few things are more appealing to a man than that.

7. Making love requires connection.
Girlfriends are one thing. Another example is having sex. To make love, you must be connected to the other person.

The key is to pay attention to both him and what you're doing at any given time. Examine each other's eyes. Tell him how pleased he makes you feel by whispering in his ear.

8. Demonstrate zeal

It may surprise you to hear that making love to a guy may also be romantic. Not only ladies like a good old-fashioned romance now and again. Making an effort to be romantic with him would be much appreciated.

Rewarding him with a great supper may also make him feel cherished and valued, so don't forget to thank him.

9. Make the setting great.

Candles, flowers, music, and mood lighting are all clichés for a reason. They do their job. Individuals, on the other hand, are prone to being engaged in what they believe to be clichéd relationships. The perfect love tale. But keep in mind that you two are in a relationship, so employ common sense. No two persons are the same. Why should you obey the rules? Why not create your own relationship on your own terms?

If you both find art appealing, try to plan a date at an artistic place before going home to make it lovely. If you and your lover like playing video games, plan a night of sex and naked gaming.

Take part in activities together and see how romantic it gets. It offers a level of common interest that allows for a deeper level of connection.

10. Give him compliments.

Make sure to compliment him since men may be just as insecure as women, especially when it comes to sex. Tell him how handsome and seductive he is, how much he attracts you, and other complimentary things. He'll feel fantastic and gain confidence in the sack as a consequence.

CHAPTER 3

11. Oral, oral, oral!

True, oral sex is a risk-free alternative. Oral sex is one of the best ways to excite his interest, yet it's easy to get into a rut and stop bothering.

Your boyfriend's delight from oral sex is well worth the fun and happiness it may bring. It's a win-win scenario since he will undoubtedly return the favor if you do it often!

12. Excited massaging, caressing, and touching

Isn't simply reading it a turn on? Go all out with your companion! Hug him and stuff his face anywhere you want.

Feel his arms, penis, and chest with your touch as he melts into you! Be a fighter!

13. novel approaches of make love to a man

When it comes to making love to a male, there are no hard and fast rules. In fact, mixing things up might keep your sexual life from becoming monotonous. There are several techniques and strategies to try. It all boils down to trying, learning, and taking chances.

14. Identify and build on his interests.

All men are not created equal. Some men like lace, while others consider that lingerie is OK but enjoy the act of undressing. Some individuals despite heels, while others like them. A flowery fragrance, for example, has the potential to alter.

Let's say he likes see-through underwear but is especially fond of the aroma of cherries. Let's claim he enjoys seeing you get fired up. You understand what has to be done.

Enjoy the process, and he will notice because he will understand why you did it. It will show him your want to please him as well as your interest in what he has to say.

15. Take on additional responsibilities.

Get your hands on a copy of Kama Sutra's sex handbook. There are hundreds of unique and entertaining sex positions to try, however some may need considerable flexibility.

Some will surely provide him with incredible, deep orgasms beyond anything he has ever experienced!

CHAPTER 4

16. Take it somewhere else.

Don't confine your sexual activity to the confines of your house. The outer world may be perilous. Outdoor sexual experiences are spontaneous, a touch nasty, and a lot of fun.

Choose a secluded location and just go for it the next time you're out and about and the need strikes! Simply keep an eye out for detection!

17. Get some edgy underwear.

Your lover will always appreciate the effort you put into looking well. Why not invest a little money on some highly lovely lingerie that will make his eyes jump instead of wearing those aged, gray granny panties?

18 Make him a strip.

He'll be drawn to a sensual striptease like never before, producing sexual tension and expectation. If you're nervous, choose the most flattering light, pretend to be alone, and wear your sexiest undergarments to increase your confidence. You'll be moving in the most seductive ways before you realize it!

19. Teach a man how to make love to him by giving him the lapdance.

Give him a lovely present with a passionate lapdance when he least expects it. Take a seat, put on some appropriate music, and get started. Understanding your own body's attractiveness and allure is part of learning how to make love to a man.

20. Pick at him

It is not essential to begin having intercourse right away. Spend some time utilizing foreplay to build tension and heighten desire.

If his hands begin to wander, give him a sweet kiss and gently push them away. Give him a little touch and then let go. Continue doing so until the temperature becomes too high to prevent the inevitable.

CHAPTER 5

21. Make him wait

You should make him wait if you want to pique his interest. This strategy works particularly well when you're just starting on dates, but it may also be used throughout a relationship.

Inform him that you will not be seeing him for a long time and that you will be taking a break from having sex. Allow him to wait with anticipation when the days pass and you can return to bed together.

22. Realize his dream

Find out what his sexual desires are and act them out. This might vary from acting as strangers at a bar to dressing as a nurse. We promise that you will grant all of his requests!

23. Alter your demeanor from courteous to evil.

Talking trash is a great way to get down and dirty under the covers. If you're not sure where to begin, go with caution at first. "It feels so good," "I'm getting so wet from you." If he gets into it, you may let your imagination go wild!

Dirty chat is an essential part of making love, not only for booty thumping. To explain how amazing something feels to him, use "naughty" terminology. Inform him that you want him to screw you hard or else you would force him to come to you. He'll love it and will make every attempt to improve the experience for you in return.

24. Tell him about your objectives and interests.

Remember how you wanted to know how to make love to a guy? Don't just say cruel things to have an orgasm. Make contact with him by chatting to him.
Express your love for the feel of his hands on your breasts. Tell him you love it when he holds your waist and pulls you in. Begin slowly and gradually increase your level of difficulty.

Certain things are just plain obvious. For example, guide him to the region on your neck where you like his kisses. Instead of asking, show him; he'll understand.

25. Have fun, both of you, without constraint.

Because making love to a man nowadays is more about connecting than having sex, women are often shy during the act.
The key is to stop thinking and start living in the present moment. Take note of what he's doing and surrender. Concentrate on and pursue your objectives. You should admire both the performance and yourself. Make him feel like you're the only woman he'll ever want, and then watch as he treats you like you're the only guy he'll ever want.

CHAPTER 6

26. Watching a pornographic movie with someone may teach you both how to make out with a man.

Why not get in on the fun? The majority of guys watch porn with or without their girlfriend. Watching porn together might be a great turn-on for you both.

Since having sex is all about trying new things, why not go to the nearest sex shop and see what's on offer? With so many sex toys available, you're certain to find something you both like to spice up your sex life.

If it is too much for you, you may look about and buy online.

27. Make more of it

The more you have, the more you will learn about each other. Then do that as frequently as you can!

Set out an hour each day to spend time in bed together, even if it seems like a chore at first. Even just lying in bed together and enjoying each other's company may result in more frequent sexual experiences.

28. Self-assurance is essential.

When it comes to making love to a man or anything else, confidence is crucial. If you try something and it doesn't work, believe in yourself!

Be confident if he makes a move that does not seem to be moving you in the direction you want!

Use your sexy smile and the eyes that make him drool as you change your stance. He won't care or even notice.

29. Experiment with sensuality!

Life is too short to continually follow the missionary sex position craze. We all have nasty, sexual impulses that we are uncomfortable sharing or trying in real life since we are all human.

But how can you two enjoy making love if you're not willing to take a little step into the unknown?

30. Make sure you're having fun as well. Telling him what you enjoy and what makes you tick can let him see that you're doing a good job, so do it! Allow him to witness you having fun!

All that matters is that you both learn efficient communication strategies in bed, and you will only become better at making love to each other with time.

CHAPTER 7

31. Be grateful for your naked body

Women who are happy in terms of sex are self-assured in their physical attractiveness. They believe they are beautiful and strong. Maintain a favorable attitude about your body. When a woman looks at herself, her gaze frequently finds her difficult places, and she brings those feelings into the bedroom. As her partner caresses her thighs, she normally thinks.

32. Check in with yourself to feel more at ease in your own skin.

Make it a practice to say body-positive affirmations. Take notice of all the attractive girls in your local proximity, representing a variety of body shapes, the next time you're in the supermarket or the gym. Remember that there is no one ideal. Next, ask your partner what he likes about your body and write it down. Review the list every morning. Finally, compliment yourself. Stand naked in front of the mirror at least once a week, if not every day, and focus on your greatest features, such as your firm buttocks, wonderful breasts, and toned arms. Feel each component and shout out your favorite feature. This will validate and support your feelings.

33. Flirt and caress

Yes, it's overkill, but it works quite well. This is because your desire for something intensifies when you tell yourself that you can't have it. This is also true in the bedroom, especially if you and your partner have been dating for a long time and sex is second nature to you. Instead of focusing on the result, learn to embrace the pleasure of sex. Tease both your spouse and yourself. Remove your clothing, dim the lights, and take turns studying each other's bodies.

34. Incorporate a few bends

It's easy to be lazy in bed. But you two deserve more credit. You will not get energy from your relationship until you put any into it.

Dopamine, a neurotransmitter required for sexual desire, may be created in the brain via fresh and exciting activities. If you take a risk outside of the bedroom, your dopamine levels and sex drive may skyrocket. When you're doing something new and fresh together, it's simpler to revisit that first passionate moment when you couldn't get enough of one other.

35. Tell your partner how to make you happy. Men want to be your knight in shining armor when it comes to sex; they want you to tell them what feels good. Having him see what makes you happy might be beneficial to both of you. Place your hand over his and tell him how to touch you, including how much pressure to apply. When you're ready to introduce some sex toys or go on to oral sex, say something. In this way, he can only discover what works for you.

CHAPTER 8

36. Adjust your timetable

Being anxious makes it difficult to feel sexy. When a woman is constantly stressed, her body produces more oxytocin, a hormone that counteracts the effects of the sex hormone testosterone. As a result, your libido plummets. Activities that enable you to get away from your hectic daily routine may help you refill your sexual vitality. When you're comfortable and confident in your talents, sex will become more feasible.

37. Be self-assured and make the first move.

A recent study found that a woman's marital pleasure was most strongly influenced by her husband's emotional participation. You're happy when you and your partner spend quality time together. When you're disengaged, your sexual life and relationship deteriorate. To be inspired to make love, you must feel connected to him, and he often needs sex to do so.

How can the deadlock be broken? Take the first step. Say something as simple as "thank you" for the little pleasures in life. When you express your gratitude to him, he becomes quite attached to you. In response, he'll start becoming what you need again, and you'll be much more motivated to want him back.

38. Take part in an intriguing activity.

You may be surprised to find that having fun and laughing together enhances your chances of having sex later on. Similar to when you first fell in love, there will be a connection between you two that generates feel-good neurotransmitters.

39. Show the oil

On instances when life has been too hectic and we haven't made time for sex, provide a massage with candles and oils. It will help you both relax, and the sensitive, intimate touch will eventually lead to kissing and sex. It provides the perfect setting for a sensual, slower-paced night when you might otherwise be "too tired."

40. Exercise

If you need more reason to exercise, consider how it may enhance your sex life. In addition to the body, it stimulates the brain and neurological system. Exercise improves blood flow to all regions of the body, strengthens the cardiovascular system, and stimulates circulation. It also enhances your mood by reducing stress and increasing your self-esteem. After working out, you feel pleased and successful. When you do it regularly, it provides you with a feeling of self-worth.

Exercise also helps you tune out the outer world and tune into your body. Yoga and weightlifting, which require you to pay attention to your form and muscles, are especially useful for this. Because you are completely focused on yourself and are aware of every action, you are in a more sensual state.

Conclusion

A deep and personal connection with a man requires more than simply sexual intimacy; emotional, mental, and physical aspects are all crucial. Communication is vital because it fosters understanding and trust. Begin by having open talks about your preferences, limitations, and desires.

Setting the tone is critical; make the place pleasant and romantic. Pay close attention to his recommendations and needs. Kissing, touching, and exploring each other's bodies may heighten the sense of foreplay, which is essential. Communication is maintained during intimacy to ensure that both individuals are comfortable and enjoying the encounter.

Remember that there is no one-size-fits-all solution. Because each man is unique, it is critical to pay attention to what he desires. Continue to express affection and connection after intercourse to deepen the emotional bond. Mutual respect and trust are the foundations of a good physical relationship.

The last word on kissing a man

Making love is more difficult than having sex. Making love implies that you and your partner have an intimacy—a connection. Making love is an extension of it. It's a means for you two to express themselves.

Without hesitation, give in and leave your inhibitions at the door.

www.ingramcontent.com/pod-product-compliance
Lightning Source LLC
Chambersburg PA
CBHW070749260726
48660CB00007B/3028